Cancer

MW01131062

A Beginner's Step-by-Step Guide With a Sample 7-Day Meal Plan

Disclaimer

By reading this disclaimer, you are accepting the terms of the disclaimer in full. If you disagree with this disclaimer, please do not read the book. The content in this book is provided for informational and educational purposes only. This book is not intended to be a substitute for the original work of this diet plan. At most, this book is intended to be beginner's supplement to the original work for this diet plan and never act as a direct substitute. This book, is an overview, review, and commentary of the facts of that diet plan.

All product names, diet plans, or names used in this book are for identification purposes only and are property of their respective owners. Use of these names does not imply endorsement. All other trademarks cited herein are property of their respective owners.

None of the information in this book should be accepted as independent medical or other professional advice.

The information in the books has been compiled from various sources that are deemed reliable. It has been analyzed and summarized to the best of the Author's ability, knowledge, and belief. However, the Author cannot guarantee the accuracy and thus should not be held liable for any errors.

You acknowledge and agree that the Author of this book will not be held liable for any damages,

Table of Contents

Introduction

Thank you for downloading this guide.
In the 1950s, a Japanese educator, lawyer, and natural food advocate named George Ohsawa believed that there is a treatment for any debilitating or chronic disease with the right kind of food. His research showed that women, challenged by cancer, may lessen the risk of suffering a relapse with a diet regimen he prepared. Even his student and protégée Michio Kushi did several seminars in the United States about a dietary regimen composed of a low-fat, but high-complex carbohydrate diet can help alleviate the progression of cancer. The goal of the diet is to eat healthier food that will make you stronger to fight cancer.

Would it be a better option to aid the medical treatments that leave you skinny and lethargic? This healthy option is called the Cancer Macrobiotic Diet.

In the **Cancer Macrobiotic Diet**, you will discover...

- The origins, advocates of the diet and how you can incorporate their belief that all-natural food is beneficial to your new eating lifestyle.

- The amazing benefits of this diet and at the same time, learn what the diet lacks so you can replenish the lost vitamins in your body.

- What foods to eat and what to avoid when you begin this diet.

- Easy to prepare recipes through the use of allowed food groups.

- A 7-Day diet plan that is low in fat and high in carbohydrates.

Chapter 1: Cancer Macrobiotic Diet in a Nutshell

The Cancer Macrobiotic Diet is a dietary regimen that is for prevention and treatment for several diseases. It also has philosophical importance as well. To maximize this kind of diet, one should still undergo some physical activities to aid the many side effects coming from radiation or chemotherapy sessions. Note: do as your physician if this diet may be beneficial to your needs as a cancer patient. Modifying your dietary intake of food is still important and self-medication or treatments you are doing should be about your disease.

In the Cancer Macrobiotic diet, vegetables consumed with a daily 30% ratio. Intake of beans is consumed with 10%, and whole grains, on the other hand, must have the entire 60%. Yes, you may still consume fish if you are not on a strict diet since the protein, iron, and other vitamins are still needed by your body. Allot at least one day a week where you may have fish as part of your lunch or dinner.

Several reports by the American Institute for Cancer Research have indicated that the risk of having cancer is lessened by 20% by consuming fruits, whole grains, and vegetables daily. With this in mind, preparing one's self to eat healthier now that cancer has started should begin with the foods to avoid and to eat. Given the food category ratio, you may opt to consume more whole grains than beans. A study showed by the World Cancer Research Fund in 1997 explained that the consumption increase of whole-grain foods showed a decrease of 20% of cancer cases worldwide.

Chapter 2: Macrobiotic Diet's Benefits and Deficiencies

At the start of cancer, you need a plan not to lose weight but rather, keep your body's immunity levels strong. While a macrobiotic diet does not promote itself as a weight loss regime, you may lose weight in the process due to certain food group restraints. The Macrobiotic diet lowers the risk for cancer due to the high amount of antioxidants, fiber and other micronutrients present. It is important to know how beneficial that you consume more food that will treat your illness. On the downside, there are some vitamins and minerals that you will miss eating. It is advisable to search for alternative food that provides the nutrition your body needs.

Note: Even though the Vitamin deficiencies may be given several alternatives, your illness may have contraindications from the medicines you are taking. To make sure you are cleared to eat this food, consult with your doctor at the beginning of this diet.

Benefits of the Macrobiotic Diet
- It helps balance your body's yin and yang through consuming natural food rather than fast food joints that contain artificial flavors.

- It helps lessen the risk of diabetes, heart disease, and chronic diseases, and cancer.
- Promotes better digestion by eating slowly and choosing fibrous food than commercialized processed food.
- Beneficial for weight reduction.
- Slows down the aging process due to food which is high in antioxidants.

Deficiencies found in the diet

This particular diet may provide certain vitamin deficiencies from Vitamin B12, calcium, and Vitamin D. The solution is to take supplements or increase the intake of vegan and vegetarian-friendly dairy and vegetables that are known to be rich in them. You still need Vitamin B-12 in your body since it helps in the formation of red blood cells. Furthermore, you need it to protect your nervous system and provide you with energy.

Rich in Vitamin B12: Dairy
- Coconut milk
- Almond milk
- Soymilk
- Yogurt
- Nutritional yeast
- Cottage cheese
- Vanilla ice cream

Rich in Calcium:
- Sesame Seeds
- Tofu
- Broccoli
- Okra
- Cabbage
- Rice
- Soya

Rich in Vitamin D:
- Mushrooms
- Cereals
- Almond Milk
- Orange juice
- Rice milk
- Vegan milk
- Soy yogurt

Chapter 3: Food to Avoid and Consume in a Cancer Macrobiotic Diet

Be mindful of the following food that you are allowed to eat for the Cancer Macrobiotic diet as well as those that you cannot eat. The reasons may vary depending on the illness, age, or dietary requirements. In general, the macrobiotic diet is suitable for vegans and vegetarians who are challenged with a specific illness.

Food to Avoid
- Red meat
- Poultry
- Dairy
- Eggs
- Processed food

Food to Consume

- All vegetables
- Rice and Pasta noodles
- All fruits
- Nuts

- Drinks
  Almond milk
  Coconut water
  Lemon juice
  Lime juice
  Orange juice

White wine (shoyu)

- Spices & Herbs
  Basil
  Bay leaf
  Black pepper
  Cardamom
  Cayenne pepper
  Chili powder
  Cinnamon
  Dill
  Garlic salt
  Chili flakes
  Garlic powder
  Nutmeg
  Rosemary
  Onion powder

- Bakery-Related
  Panko bread crumbs
  Whole grain bread
  Rye
  Gluten-Free Tortilla
  Spelt

- Others
  Kimchi
  Brown rice
  Lentils
  Lima beans
  Hemp powder
  Red kidney beans
  Corn-based snacks
  Stevia sweetener

White kidney beans
Sweet corn

- Dairy
  Unsalted butter
  Cheddar cheese
  Ghee
  Unsalted margarine

- Cereals
  Quinoa
  Quick oats
  Steel oats

- Condiments

  Apple cider vinegar
  Soy sauce (tamari)
  Yellow mustard
  Sriracha
  Sesame oil
  Chipotle paste
  Marinara pasta sauce
  Coconut amino
  Coconut oil
  Dijon mustard
  Extra virgin oil
  Avocado oil
  Balsamic vinegar
  Canola oil
  Flaxseed oil
  Grapeseed oil
  Salsa

- Seafood
  Mackerel
  Tuna
  Salmon
  Tilapia
  Trout

Chapter 4: Cancer Macrobiotic Diet Meal Plan – Day 1

Here are recommended recipes for you that have low calories but high carbohydrates. These recipes are easy to prepare and may be stored in the refrigerator or freezer for the next day. The goal is to keep you satiated, and energetic which you will be receiving from the carbohydrates.

Breakfast: Macrobiotic Apple and Oats Porridge

Serves: 4
Calories: 154/serving
Protein: 1.1g
Fat: 0.6g
Carbohydrates: 40.8 g

Ingredients:
- 5 cups apples (cubed)
- Stevia sweetener (to taste)
- Water
- Cardamom
- 1 Lemon
- Raisins (for toppings)

Instructions:
1. Cook oats in a small pan until done.

2. Add the ingredients and mix to combine in medium to low heat.
3. As the apples soften, serve on top of the oats.

Lunch: Arugula and Mushroom Salad

Serves: 2
Calories: 104/serving
Protein: 11g
Fat: 2g
Carbohydrates: 16.5g

Ingredients:
- 5 oz. arugula washed
- 1 lb. fresh mushrooms
- ¼ teaspoon shoyu
- ½ red onion
- Tofu cheese*
- 1/2 teaspoon salt
- 1 tablespoon olive oil
- 1 tablespoon mirin

Tofu Cheese Ingredients:
- ⅛ cup umeboshi vinegar
- ½ firm tofu

Instructions:
1. In a small bowl, add the rinsed tofu; crumble and pour in the vinegar.
2. In a medium-sized bowl add the shoyu, tofu cheese, red onions, salt, olive oil, and mirin; mix to combine.
3. Add in the arugula and toss to combine with the dressing.
4. Serve on a plate and enjoy!

Dinner: Garbanzo-Kale & Butternut Squash Burger

Serves: 4
Calories: 397 /serving
Protein: 13.6g
Fat: 11.1g
Carbohydrates: 63.1g

Ingredients:
- 1/2 cup brown rice
- 1/2 cup quinoa

Beetroot burger
- 2 cups kale
- 1 teaspoon paprika
- 1 cup butternut squash (chopped)
- 1/2 cup sauerkraut bottled
- 3/4 cup garbanzo beans
- 2 tablespoon coconut oil
- 1 teaspoon of sea salt

Instructions:
1. In a pan, add the quinoa and water; bring to boil and cook for 20 minutes.
2. In a chopping board, slice the kale, butternut squash, and transfer to a small bowl.
3. Add the paprika, garbanzo beans, sea salt, and coconut oil; sauté mixture until vegetables soften.

4. Prepare the burger by making balls; flatten burger and fry until done.
5. Serve on a plate and enjoy!

Chapter 5: Cancer Macrobiotic Diet Meal Plan – Day 2

Breakfast: Berry-Lemon Mochi Waffles
Serves: 2
Calories: 145/serving
Protein: 3g
Fat: 11.9g
Carbohydrates: 9.4g

Ingredients:
- 2 tablespoons strawberry and lemon sauce
- ¼ cup toasted pine nuts
- 1 teaspoon lemon (zest)
- 4 mint leaves (for topping)
- 1 lb. mochi

Instructions:
1. On a cutting board, uniformly slice the mochi into ¼ strips.
2. Prepare a non-stick waffle maker and cook the mochi strips until golden brown.
3. Transfer waffles on a serving plate; garnish with strawberry and lemon sauce and top with mint leaves.

Lunch – Cyprian Cheese and Greens Salad with Pesto Dressing

Serves: 4/serving
Calories: 640/serving
Protein: 5.1g
Fat: 62.7
Carbohydrates: 21.1g

Ingredients:

Salad
- 2 heads lettuce (large)
- 1/4 bulb fennel
- 2 cucumbers
- 1 avocado
- ¼ cup toasted almonds
- 1 packet halloumi/vegan cheese
- ¼ cup basil leaves
- 1/8 cup dill
- Black peppercorns
- 2 tablespoon lemon juice
- Olive oil

Pesto Sauce:
- 1 cup toasted almonds
- 1 lemon
- 1/2 cup arugula
- 1 cup olive oil

Instructions:

1. In a food processor, prepare the pesto sauce by adding all ingredients together; blend to smoothen; season with lemon juice, pepper, and salt to taste.
2. In a large salad bowl, add the herbs and remaining vegetables.
3. Transfer pesto sauce in a small bowl, and serve with the salad.
4. In a pan, prepare the halloumi by frying until crunchy at the sides; serve salad greens and pesto sauce.

Dinner – Hearty Cauliflower-Garbanzo Stew

Serves: 4
Calories: 279/serving
Protein: 13.2g
Fat: 3g
Carbohydrates: 38.6g

Ingredients:
- 1 medium carrot
- 1 can diced tomatoes
- Salt and pepper (to taste)
- Parsley, chopped, for serving
- 1 lemon, juiced for serving
- 1 cup farro grains
- 1 small yellow onion
- Olive oil
- 1/2 teaspoon paprika
- 2 cups garbanzos
- 3 cloves garlic
- 2 teaspoons cumin
- 1/2 teaspoon cinnamon
- 2 cups vegetable broth
- 1 head cauliflower
- 1/8 teaspoon cayenne

Instructions:

1. In a medium-sized pan, sauté the garlic, onions, and olive oil, paprika, cayenne, and cinnamon for two minutes.
2. In a pot, boil garbanzos and cauliflower until soft.
3. Serve in a bowl and season with lemon juice, pepper and salt to taste; top with parsley, and farro.

Chapter 6: Cancer Macrobiotic Diet Meal Plan: Day 3

Breakfast: Vietnamese Early Rush Baguette

Serves: 4
Calories: 484/serving
Protein: 12.1g
Fat: 16g
Carbohydrates: 72g

Ingredients:

For the tofu
- 2 tablespoons maple syrup
- 3 tablespoons lime juice
- 2 tablespoons coconut aminos
- 1 block extra-firm tofu
- 1 clove garlic
- 1 tablespoon smoked paprika

For the sandwich
- 2 scallions
- ½ cup vegan mayo
- 4 sliced fresh baguettes
- 1/8 cup fresh cilantro

For the pickles
- 2 small carrots
- 1 small radish
- ¼ cup of rice vinegar

- ¼ cup white wine vinegar
- Salt to taste

Instructions:
For the tofu

1. Drain excess liquid from tofu, slice into baguette-sized portions and place in a medium-sized bowl; add the ingredients for the marinade, set aside from 20 minutes.
2. Transfer marinated tofu slices to a grilling pan; grill about 4 minutes per side.
3. Prepare bottle vegan mayo; set aside for later.

For the pickles

1. In a medium-sized bowl, add salt, and turmeric, and salt.
2. Add radish, and julienned carrots; allow to marinate for 15 minutes or longer.
3. Prepare the baguettes, spread vegan mayo on top.
4. Assemble the hearty breakfast veggie baguette by layering the pickled vegetables, and tofu slices.
5. Serve on a plate and top with extra tomato slices and cilantro for garnishing.

Lunch: Garlic-Cashews Red Pasta

Serves: 4
Calories: 604/serving
Protein: 18.1g
Fat: 31.1g
Carbohydrates: 74.7g

Ingredients:

- 1 lb. pasta
- 1/2 cup cashews, ground into a powder
- 1/2 cup vegan cream cheese
- 1/4 cup extra-virgin olive oil (reserve for drizzling)
- 1 tablespoon tomato paste, optional
- 1 red bell pepper
- 4 cloves garlic
- Black pepper, to Taste
- Salt, to Taste

Instructions:

1. Prepare an aluminum foil and lay the garlic cloves; drizzle with olive oil and bake at 350 degrees Fahrenheit for 30 minutes. Increase oven temperature to 450 degrees Fahrenheit to roast red peppers; cook for 30 minutes until blackened.
2. In a food processor, add the Vegan cream cheese, oil, red pepper, cashew powder, tomato paste, pepper, and salt; blend until smooth.

Dinner – Macrobiotic Bowl Medley

Serves: 4
Calories: 556 /serving
Protein: 28.1g
Fat: 3.3g
Carbohydrates: 107.5g

Ingredients:
For the Bowl
- 1/2 cup brown rice
- 3 cup chard, roughly chopped
- 1 cup squash, diced
- 1 cup broccoli florets
- 1 cup black beans
- 1 oz. kombu
- 1/2 cup sauerkraut, chopped

For the Sauce
- 2 tablespoon sesame tahini
- 2 tablespoon sodium tamari
- 1 clove garlic
- 1 tablespoon ginger
- 1 lime, juiced

Instructions:
For the Bowl
1. Bring 1 cup of water to a boil for the rice. Once boiling, add rice, return to boil, cover then reduce heat and simmer 40 minutes. Remove from heat and allow to

sit covered an additional 10 minutes then fluff with a fork.

2. Thoroughly rinse and drain beans, then transfer to a pot with kombu, cover with water, bring to a boil, reduce heat and simmer 15-20 minutes then drain and rinse.

3. Place a steamer basket in a pot with water and bring to a boil.

4. Add broccoli, cover and steam 4-5 minutes then remove, keeping water in the pot.

5. Add squash, cover and steam 4-5 minutes then remove, keeping water in the pot.

6. Add chard, cover and steam 3-4 minutes, then remove.

7. Serve on a plate and enjoy!

Chapter 7: Cancer Macrobiotic Diet Meal Plan – Day 4

Breakfast: Asian Themed Macrobiotic Bowl

Serves: 4
Calories: 572/serving
Protein: 18.4g
Fat: 21.4g
Carbohydrates: 667 kcal

Ingredients
- 2 cups cooked quinoa
- 4 carrots
- 1 package of smoked tofu
- 1 tablespoon nutritional yeast
- 2 tablespoon coconut aminos
- 4 tablespoon of sunflower sprouts
- 2 tablespoon of fermented vegetables
- 1 cup of shiitake mushrooms
- 1 avocado
- 2 tablespoon hemp seeds
- 2-3 cooked beets
- Coconut oil cooking spray

Dressing
- 2 tablespoon miso paste
- 1 tablespoon tahini
- 1 clove garlic, crushed
- 1 tablespoon olive oil
- ½ lime, juiced
- 3 tablespoon of water

Instructions:
1. First, roast the carrots in the oven at 400 degrees for 30-40 minutes. Washed them, trim, and spray in coconut oil; when they are cooked, set aside till you are ready to assemble the Buddha bowl.
2. Make the dressing by combining all of the dressing ingredients in a medium-size bowl. If the dressing appears lumpy, add more water.
3. To build the bowl, put the quinoa on the bottom and then arrange the vegetables on top, sprinkle the bowls with hemp seeds and drizzle the dressing over top.
4. Now serve and enjoy!

Lunch: Italian Sweet Pepper-Tomato Pasta

Serves: 2
Calories: 561/serving
Protein: 15.2g
Fat: 24.4g
Carbohydrates: 73.4g

Ingredients:
- 2 small red onions, diced
- 3 tablespoon olive oil
- 3/4 teaspoon garlic powder
- 1 vegetable stock cube
- 1/2 teaspoon sea salt
- 1 teaspoon cumin
- 1/4 teaspoon cinnamon
- 1 tablespoon dried basil
- 1 cup of fresh parsley
- 1 tablespoon dried oregano
- 2 sprigs fresh oregano
- 1/2 black pepper
- 1 cup canned Roma tomatoes
- 1 tablespoon dried cilantro
- 2 red tomatoes, chopped
- 1 cup baby sweet peppers
- ½ lb. pasta

Instructions:

1. In a large pan, heat the olive oil for 30 seconds; add onions, spices, and vegetable stock.
2. Incorporate the tomatoes, herbs, and pepper; simmer for about 15 minutes.
3. Once tomatoes are soft, mash with a fork or transfer to a food processor.
4. In the same pan, add water and pasta; cook until al dente.
5. Serve on a plate, top with extra basil leaf garnishing.

Dinner – Moroccan Rice Noodle Curry Soup

Serves: 4
Total Calories: 685/serving
Protein: 9.3g
Fat: 57.7g
Carbohydrates: 40.8g

Ingredients

- 8 oz. rice noodles
- 1 tablespoon ginger
- 1 cup of frozen green beans
- 1 red bell pepper
- 1 tablespoon coconut oil
- 1/3 cup diced white onion
- 2 (15 oz.) cans coconut milk
- 1 1/2 teaspoon lime juice
- 2 carrots
- 3 cloves garlic
- 1 cup vegetable broth
- Cilantro, fresh, for serving
- 2 1/2 tablespoons red curry paste
- 2 cups broccoli florets
- Sea salt, to taste

Instructions:

1. In a deep soup pot, add coconut oil, sauté garlic, onions, and ginger until the onions turn translucent.
2. Add coconut milk and stir in the curry paste,

3. Add bell peppers, vegetable broth, carrots, and lime juice; boil and simmer at medium to low heat for 15 minutes.
4. In a separate pot, cook rice noodles according to instructions found in the package.
5. Use the same soup pot, add the frozen green beans, broccoli; cook until tender for 10 minutes.
6. To serve, ladle soup in a bowl, add the cooked rice noodles and garnish with cilantro; sprinkle sea salt to taste.

Chapter 8: Cancer Macrobiotic Diet Meal Plan: Day 5

Breakfast: Broccoli-Kale with Avocado Toppings Rice Bowl

Serves: 2
Total Calories: 327/serving
Protein: 8.4g
Fat: 11.2g
Carbohydrates: 50g

Ingredients:
- 1/2 avocado
- 2 cups kale
- 1 cup broccoli florets
- 1/2 cup cooked brown rice
- 1 teaspoon plum vinegar
- 2 teaspoon tamari
- Sea salt, to taste

Instructions:
1. In a small pot, simmer broccoli florets, and kale in about 3 tablespoons of water; cook for 2 minutes.
2. Add tamari, vinegar, and cooked brown rice; stir to combine.
3. Transfer pot contents into a medium-sized bowl and top with sliced avocado; sprinkle a dash of sea salt to taste.

Lunch – Tofu Noodle Bowl in Citrusy Soy Sauce

Serves: 2
Calories: 469/serving
Protein: 22.7g
Fat: 6.3g
Carbohydrates: 89g

Ingredients:
For Citrusy Soy sauce
- 4 teaspoons maple syrup
- 2 teaspoons garlic chili sauce
- 2 limes (juice)
- 1/4 cup tamari
- 1/2 teaspoon garlic powder
- 2 minced scallions
- ¼ cup of water

For Tofu noodles
- 1 block extra-firm tofu
- 4 scallions, crosswise halved
- 16 oz. buckwheat noodles
- 2 teaspoons garlic chili sauce
- 2 teaspoons tamari
- 2 cups broccoli florets
- 2 small julienned cucumbers

Instructions:
1. Prepare the citrusy soy sauce by whisking all ingredients in a small bowl; set aside for 15 minutes.

2. To make tofu noodles, use a skillet to sauté tamari, garlic chili sauce, and broccoli until softened.
3. Transfer noodles in a medium-sized bowl and top with broccoli, tofu, cucumber, and scallions; pour citrusy soy sauce on top.

Dinner – Lemon Drop Cannellini Bean Soup

Serves: 6
Total Calories: 536/serving
Protein: 31.2g
Fat: 10.3g
Carbohydrates: 83.2g

Ingredients:

- 2 cans cannellini beans
- 4 cups vegetable broth
- 2 tablespoon olive oil
- 1 finely chopped yellow onion
- 2 finely chopped large carrots
- 1 teaspoon kosher salt
- 1 teaspoon freshly cracked black pepper
- 4 minced garlic cloves
- 1 can chickpeas
- 3 teaspoon finely chopped fresh rosemary
- 1 bunch roughly chopped spinach
- 1 lemon (zest and juice)
- 1/3 cup nutritional yeast

Instructions:

1. In a blender, combine 1 cup of broth, and 1 cup cannellini beans; blend until smooth then set aside.
2. In a large stockpot, heat oil over medium heat; add carrots, and onions until softened.

3. Add remaining cannellini beans, rosemary, and chickpeas; stir to combine for one minute.
4. Boil 3 cups broth, bean mixture, and chopped spinach for 25 minutes or until thick.
5. Stir in juice and zest of lemon, and sprinkle in the nutritional yeast.
6. Ladle hearty soup in 6 individual bowls; add with black pepper and rosemary for garnish.

Chapter 9: Cancer Macrobiotic Diet Meal Plan: Day 6

Breakfast – Vegetable Pasta in Avocado Sauce

Serves: 4
Total Calories: 325/serving
Protein: 6.4g
Fat: 23.6g
Carbohydrates: 26.1g

Ingredients:

Zucchini Pasta
- 2 zucchini
- 3 cups red and yellow cherry tomatoes
- 4 oz. pasta

Avocado Sauce
- 1/2 cup fresh parsley
- 1 tablespoon miso paste
- 1 garlic clove
- 1 avocado
- 1/4 cup olive oil
- 4 green onions
- 1/2 teaspoon salt
- 1 lemon (juiced)
- Ground pepper to taste

Instructions:
1. To make the avocado sauce, use a blender to pulse all ingredients until smooth; set aside.

2. In a large skillet over high heat, drizzle olive oil and cook cherry tomatoes until skin loosens; season with ground pepper and salt.
3. In the same skillet, add the zucchini, and avocado sauce; toss to combine.
4. To serve, season with ground pepper and salt to taste; garnish with extra tomatoes.

Lunch - Grilled Macrobiotic Bowl with Stir Fry Broccoli, Onions and Carrots

Serves: 4
Total Calories: 340/serving (first recipe)
117/serving (second recipe)
Protein: 9.7g (first recipe) 3g (second recipe)
Fat: 18.6g (first recipe) 5g (second recipe)
Carbohydrates: 36.2g (first recipe) 17.3g (second recipe)

Ingredients
- 2 tablespoon garlic, minced
- 2 tablespoon olive oil
- 1/2 cup adzuki beans cooked
- 1/2 cup sauerkraut
- 1 cup quinoa
- 1/2 cup cubed butternut squash
- 1 tablespoon dulse flakes
- 1 1/2 cup baby kale
- 1 tablespoon toasted pumpkin seeds
- Salt and pepper to taste

Garlic Cashew Creme
- 3 cloves garlic
- 1/2 cup raw cashews
- 1 lemon (juice)
- 1/2 teaspoon sea salt

Instructions:
Bowl
1. Add the butternut in a large glass bowl to pre-cook for 2 minutes.

2. On the grill, spread some olive oil and add rice, butternut, sauerkraut, greens, and beans.
3. For 5 to 7 minutes, grill on medium-high turning the ingredients frequently until cooked.
4. Sprinkle a dash of salt and pepper to taste.

Garlic Cashew Creme
1. Blend all ingredients in a high-speed blender; set aside.

Assemble bowl
1. Sprinkle dulse flakes and toasted pumpkin seeds; top with Garlic Cashew Creme

Stir Fry Broccoli, Onions and Carrots
Ingredients:
 1 teaspoon light olive oil
 1 ½ cups onion
 2 cups medium-sized carrots
 6 cups medium-sized broccoli
 2 ½-inch broccoli flowerets
 ¼ teaspoon of sea salt
 ½ cup of water
 1 tablespoon soy sauce (optional)

Instructions:
1. In a pan, heat the sesame oil to medium-high heat; add to sauté the onions.
2. Sauté the carrots, broccoli, the flowerets, then add water; season with sea salt and cover the pan to bring to a boil.
3. Lower the heat and bring to a simmer for 5 minutes.
4. Pour some soy sauce if needed.

Reminder:
1. Stir-fried vegetables, top with some pasta or rice.
2. Substitute other vegetables such as cabbage, cabbage, cauliflower, or yellow squash.
3. For additional flavor, sauté 1 tablespoon of minced ginger in the oil before adding the carrots.

Chapter 10: Cancer Macrobiotic Diet Meal Plan: Day 7

Breakfast – Banana Walnut-Maple Oatmeal
Serves: 1
Calories: 645/serving
Protein: 7.8g
Fat: 38.2g
Carbohydrates: 15.8g

Ingredients:
- 1 teaspoon pure maple syrup
- 2 tablespoon chopped walnuts
- ½ cup gluten-free rolled oats
- 2 tablespoon sun butter
- ½ cup of water
- ½ banana, sliced
- ½ cup almond milk
- A pinch of salt
- ¼ cup pumpkin puree
- ¼ teaspoon cinnamon
- Nutmeg for topping

Instructions:
1. In a small pan, bring the almond milk, oats, water, and salt to a boil; simmer for 5 minutes.
2. Remove pan from heat, add in the pumpkin puree and sun butter; stir gently to cover the oats.
3. Add the remaining ingredients such as cinnamon, and chopped walnuts.

4. Transfer oatmeal in a bowl and garnish with nutmeg powder.

Lunch – Avocado and Caesar Salad

Serves: 3
Calories: 508/serving
Protein: 42.3g
Fat: 30.5g
Carbohydrates: 26.5g

Ingredients:

- 1 head romaine hearts, washed
- 1 package of tempeh
- 1 small red onion
- 1/2 avocado (sliced)

Instruction:

1. Slice the red onion and place in a bowl.
2. Add 1/16 teaspoon of sea salt and 3 drops of umeboshi vinegar.
3. Very gently rub the salt and vinegar into the onion until you see the color deepen; set aside until you are ready to assemble your salad.
4. Wash the romaine and remove excess water using a salad spinner or cotton towel.
5. Break the lettuce into a bowl.
6. Add the red onion and the tempeh; lightly toss with your hands or wooden utensils.
7. Add fresh avocado slices and toss to coat the lettuce.

8. Drizzle a little umeboshi vinegar over the entire salad then toss to blend the ingredients.

Dinner – Hickory Tempeh, and Broccoli Roast Bowl

Serves: 1
Calories: 438/serving
Protein: 42.1g
Fat: 24.5g
Carbohydrates: 21.3g

Ingredients
- Hickory sauce (to taste)
- 1 (8 oz) tempeh block

Hickory Tempeh Instructions:
1. In a small pot, submerge the tempeh in water; place enough liquid to cover the pot.
2. Bring the small pot to a boil for 5 minutes; drain liquid.
3. On a cutting board, transfer the tempeh and slice into thick chunks.
4. Transfer tempeh chunks to a skillet, and cover it with hickory sauce; allow the sauce to marinate for 15 minutes.
5. Once done, sear the tempeh chunks for 2 minutes per side; brush once more with hickory sauce.

Ingredients:
- 1 head broccoli, cut into florets
- 1 teaspoon balsamic vinegar
- Garlic powder, to taste
- Black pepper, to taste

- Salt, to taste

Broccoli Roast Instructions:
1. Preheat your oven to 475 degrees Fahrenheit and line baking sheet with aluminum foil.
2. Place the broccoli, and smear with balsamic vinegar, salt, black pepper, and garlic powder; roast for 20 minutes until broccoli is semi-charred.

Guacamole Ingredients:
- 1/4 jalapeno pepper
- 2 tablespoons diced red onion
- 1 large avocado
- 1/4 cup diced tomatoes
- 1 tablespoon chopped cilantro
- Brown rice, for serving
- 2 teaspoons fresh lime juice
- Black pepper, to taste
- Red pepper flakes, to taste
- Salt, to taste

Instructions:
1. In a small bowl, mix all the provided ingredients; stir well to incorporate then adjust seasoning depending on your taste.

Conclusion

Thank you again for getting this guide. I'd like to thank you and congratulate you for transiting my lines from start to finish.

I hope this book was able to help you to start preparing a week's collection of recipes that uses the principle of Macrobiotics. You will notice that breakfast recipes are usually easier to prepare than lunch and dinner. It is recommended to prepare the more difficult recipes in advance and store them in your refrigerator.

For every recipe, you are provided with serving sizes, and calorie counters for your guidance. Do not be alarmed if the calories are high; under the Cancer Macrobiotic Diet, your body needs to recover from the medical treatments. The recipes serve 2 at the least for you to consume the remaining the following day. This way, your diet will not exceed your weekly budget.

I also hope that the benefits of this diet will convince you to embrace natural food to help you treat your illness. Cooking is enjoyed with the family as well however if they are in a different diet, the provided recipes may perk up the menu list.

If you found this guide helpful, please take the time to share your thoughts and post a review. It'd be greatly appreciated!
I wish you the best of luck!